I0500259

Cesarean Section

Indications and Technique

Akmal El-Mazny

Copyright © 2017 Akmal El-Mazny

All rights reserved.

CreateSpace, Charleston SC, USA

ISBN-13: 978-1548409173
ISBN-10: 1548409170

CONTENTS

INTRODUCTION

Cesarean section (CS) is defined as the delivery of a fetus through surgical incisions made through the abdominal wall (laparotomy) and the uterine wall (hysterotomy).

Currently, CS is performed for a variety of maternal indications, fetal indications, or both; the leading indications are previous CS, breech presentation, dystocia, and fetal distress.

The steps for CS includes preoperative preparation, operative procedure (laparotomy, hysterotomy, fetal delivery, uterine repair, and abdominal closure), and postoperative care.

Major sources of morbidity and mortality with CS can be related to sequelae of surgical injury, anesthetic complications, infection, and thromboembolic disease.

Decreasing the rate of primary CS and increased implementation of vaginal birth after CS are important steps of a larger movement towards decreasing the overall rate of CS.

This book provides a comprehensive review of CS, emphasizing its indications and technique, which will be of immense value for obstetricians and allied health professionals.

BACKGROUND

Cesarean section (CS) is defined as the delivery of a fetus through surgical incisions made through the abdominal wall (laparotomy) and the uterine wall (hysterotomy).

The early history of caesarean section remains shrouded in myth and is of dubious accuracy.

According to legend, Julius Caesar was born in this manner, the procedure became known as the caesarean operation.

The name of the operation is derived from a roman law known as the Lex Regia, ordering that the procedure be performed upon women dying in the last few weeks of pregnancy in the hope of saving the child.

Lex Regia turned into Lex Caesarea in about 200 B.C. where the kings became Cesars.

Initially, CS was performed to separate the mother and the fetus in an attempt to save the fetus of a moribund patient.

Key steps in reducing mortality were:

−Introduction of the transverse incision technique to minimize bleeding by Ferdinand Adolf Kehrer in 1881 is thought to be first modern CS performed.

−The introduction of uterine suturing by Max Sänger in 1882.

−Modification by Hermann Johannes Pfannenstiel in 1900.

−Extraperitoneal CS and then moving to low transverse incision by Krönig in 1912.

−Adherence to principles of asepsis.

−Anesthesia advances.

−Antibiotics.

−Blood transfusion.

This operation subsequently developed into a surgical procedure to resolve maternal or fetal complications not amenable to vaginal delivery, either for mechanical limitations or to temporize delivery for maternal or fetal benefit.

The CS has evolved from a vain attempt performed to save the fetus to one in which physician and patient both participate in the decision-making process, striving to achieve the most benefit for the patient and her unborn child.

Currently, CS is performed for a variety of fetal and maternal indications; the indications have expanded to consider the patient's wishes and preferences.

Controversy surrounds the current rates of CS in developed countries and its use for indications other than medical necessity.

RATE OF CS

From 1910-1928, the CS rate at Chicago Lying-in Hospital increased from 0.6% to 3%.

The CS rate in the US was 4.5% in 1965.

According to the National Hospital Discharge Survey, the CS rate rose from 5.5% in 1970 to 24.1% in 1986.

Fewer than 10% of mothers had a vaginal birth after CS (VBAC), and women spent an average of 5 days in the hospital for a CS and only 2.6 days for a vaginal delivery.

It was predicted that if age-specific CS rates continued at the steady pattern of increase observed since 1970, 40% of births would be by CS in the year 2000; those predictions fell short, but not by much.

The National Center for Health Statistics reported that the percentage of CS births in the US increased from 20.7% in 1996 to 32.2% in 2014.

CS rates increased for women of all ages, races/ethnic groups, and gestational ages and in all states.

Both primary and repeat CS increased.

Increases in the primary CS with no specified indication were faster than in the overall population and appear to be the result of changes in obstetric practice rather than changes in the medical risk profile or increases in maternal request.

This has occurred despite several studies that note an increased risk for neonatal and maternal mortality for all CS as well as for medically elective CS compared with vaginal births.

The decrease in total and repeat CS rates noted between 1990 and 2000 was due to a transient increase in the rate of vaginal births after CS.

The CS rate has also increased throughout the world, but rates in certain parts of the world are still substantially lower than in the US.

The CS rate is approximately 21% for the most developed regions of the world, 14% for the less developed regions, and 2% for the least developed regions.

In a 2006 publication reviewing CS rates in South America, the median rate was 33% with rates fluctuating between 28% and 75% depending on public service versus a private provider.

The authors conclude that higher rates of CS do not necessarily indicate better perinatal care and can be associated with harm.

Why the rate of CS has increased so dramatically in the US is not entirely clear.

Some reasons that may account for the increase are repeat CS, delay in childbirth and reduced parity, decrease in the rate of vaginal breech delivery, decreased perinatal mortality with CS, nonreassuring fetal heart rate testing, and fear of malpractice litigation.

In 1988, when the CS rate peaked at 24.7%, 36.3% of all CS were repeat procedures.

Although reports concerning the safety of allowing VBAC had been present since the 1960s, by 1987, fewer than 10% of women with a prior CS were attempting a vaginal delivery.

In 2003, the repeat CS rate for all women was 89.4%; the rate for low-risk women was 88.7%.

Today, low-risk women giving birth for the first time who have a CS are more likely to have a subsequent CS.

In the past decade, an increase in the percentage of births to women aged 30-50 years has occurred despite a decrease in their relative size within the population.

The CS rate for mothers aged 40-54 years in 2007 was more than twice the CS rate for mothers younger than 20 years (48% and 23%, respectively).

The risk of having a CS is higher in nulliparous patients, and, with increasing maternal age.

The risk for CS is increased secondary to medical complications such as diabetes and preeclampsia.

By 1985, almost 85% of all breech presentations (3% of term fetuses) were delivered by CS.

In 2001, a multicenter and multinational prospective study determined that the safest mode of delivery for a breech presentation was CS.

This study has been criticized for differences in the standards of care among the study centers that does not allow a standard recommendation.

The most recent recommendation from the American College of Obstetricians and Gynecologists (ACOG) regarding breech delivery is that planned vaginal delivery may be reasonable under hospital-specific protocol guidelines for both eligibility and labor management.

This may lead to a small decrease in breech delivery rates, but the overwhelming majority of cases will probably continue to be delivered by elective CS.

A cluster-randomized controlled trial reported a significant but small reduction in the rate of CS.

The benefit was driven by the effect of the intervention in low-risk pregnancies.

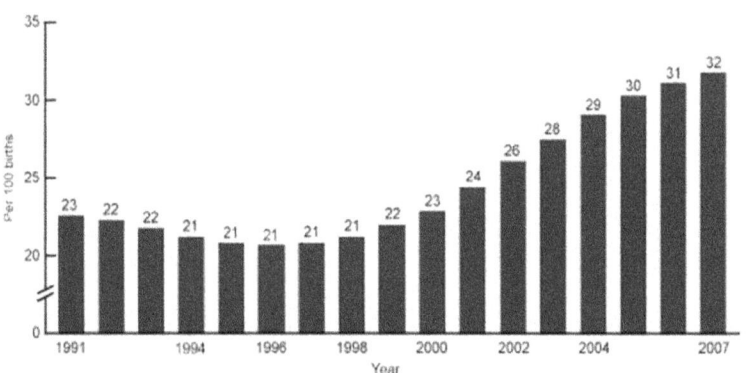

Rates of CS in US

INDICATIONS OF CS

Many indications exist for performing a CS.

In those women who are having a scheduled procedure (ie, an elective or indicated repeat, for malpresentation or placental abnormalities), the decision has already been made that the alternate of medical therapy, ie, a vaginal delivery, is least optimal.

For other patients admitted to labor and delivery, the anticipation is for a vaginal delivery.

Every patient admitted in this circumstance is admitted with the thought of a successful vaginal delivery.

However, if the patient's situation should change, a CS is performed because it is believed that outcome may be better for the fetus, the mother, or both.

A CS is performed for maternal indications, fetal indications, or both.

The leading indications for CS are previous CS, breech presentation, dystocia, and fetal distress.

These indications are responsible for 85% of all CS.

MATERNAL INDICATIONS

Maternal indications for CS include the following:

−Repeat CS.

−Obstructive lesions in the lower genital tract, including malignancies, large vulvovaginal condylomas, obstructive vaginal septa, and leiomyomas of the lower uterine segment that interfere with engagement of the fetal head.

−Pelvic abnormalities that preclude engagement or interfere with descent of the fetal presentation in labor.

Relative maternal indications include conditions in which the increasing intrathoracic pressure generated by Valsalva maneuvers could lead to maternal complications.

These include left heart valvular stenosis, dilated aortic valve root, certain cerebral arteriovenous malformations (AVMs), and recent retinal detachment.

Women who have previously undergone vaginal or perineal reparative surgery (eg, colporrhaphy or repair of major anal involvement from inflammatory bowel disease) also benefit from CS to avoid damage to the previous surgical repair.

No clear evidence supports planned CS for extreme maternal obesity.

Dystocia in labor (labor dystocia) is a very commonly cited indication for CS, but it is not specific.

Dystocia is classified as a protraction disorder or as an arrest disorder.

These can be primary or secondary disorders.

Most dystocias are caused by abnormalities of the power (uterine contractions), the passage (maternal pelvis), or the passenger (the fetus).

When a diagnosis of dystocia in labor is made, the indication should be detailed according to the previous classification (ie, primary or secondary disorder, arrest or protraction disorder, or a combination of the above).

Recently, debate has arisen over the option of elective CS delivery on maternal request (CDMR).

Evidence shows that it is reasonable to inform the pregnant woman requesting a CS of the associated risks and benefits for the current and any subsequent pregnancies.

The clinician's role should be to provide the best possible evidence-based counseling to the woman and to respect her autonomy and decision-making capabilities when considering route of delivery.

A survey of participants in the 2006 state-of-the-science conference revealed that most obstetrician/gynecologists believe that a woman has the right to CDMR, but fewer agree to perform the procedure than they did in 2006.

The 2013 ACOG Committee on Obstetric Practice and 2006 National Institutes of Health (NIH) consensus committee determined that the evidence supporting this concept was not conclusive and that more research is needed.

Both committees provided the following recommendations regarding CDMR:

– Unless there are maternal or fetal indications for CS, vaginal delivery should be recommended.

– CDMR should not be performed before 39 weeks' gestation without verifying fetal lung maturity (due to a potential risk of respiratory problems for the baby).

– CDMR is not recommended for women who want more children (due to the increased risk for placenta previa/accreta and gravid hysterectomy with each CS).

– The inavailability of effective analgesia should not be a determinant for CDMR.

The NIH consensus panel on CDMR also noted the following:

– CDMR has a potential benefit of decreased risk of hemorrhage for the mother and decreased risk of birth injuries for the baby.

– CDMR requires individualized counseling by the practitioner of the potential risks and benefits of both vaginal and CS.

FETAL INDICATIONS

Fetal indications for CS include the following:

− Situations in which neonatal morbidity and mortality could be decreased by the prevention of trauma.

− Malpresentations.

− Certain congenital malformations or skeletal disorders.

− Fetal infection.

− Prolonged acidemia.

− Maternal genital herpes infection.

− Maternal HIV infetion.

A fetus in a nonvertex presentation is at increased risk for trauma, cord prolapse, and head entrapment.

Malpresentation includes preterm breech presentations and non-frank breech term fetuses.

The decision to proceed with a CS for the term frank breech singleton fetus has been challenged.

Although most practitioners will always perform a CS in this situation, ACOG has left open the option to consider a breech delivery under the appropriate circumstances, including a practitioner experienced in the evaluation and management of labor and skilled in the delivery of the breech fetus.

Some state maternal care collaborative agencies are even implementing tools to decrease the likelihoond of CS in the instance of a breech presentation, with guidelines recommending the formation of a team in the hospital that is trained and confortable with breach and operative deliveries.

If a patient is diagnosed with a fetal malpresentation (ie, breech or transverse lie) after 36 weeks, the option for an external cephalic version is offered to try to convert the fetus to a vertex lie, thus allowing an attempt at a vaginal delivery.

An external cephalic version is usually attempted at 36-38 weeks with studies underway to establish the use of performing external cephalic version at 34 weeks' gestational age.

Ultrasonography is performed to confirm a breech presentation.

If the fetus is still in a nonvertex presentation, an IV line is started, and the baby is monitored with an external fetal heart rate monitor prior to the procedure to confirm well-being.

With a reassuring fetal heart rate tracing, the version is attempted.

An external cephalic version involves trying to externally manipulate the fetus into a vertex presentation.

This is accomplished with ultrasonographic guidance to ascertain fetal lie.

An attempt is made to manipulate the fetus through either a "forward roll" or "backward roll".

The overall chance of success is approximately 60%.

Some practitioners administer an epidural to the patient before attempting version, and others may give the patient a dose of subcutaneous terbutaline (a beta-mimetic used for tocolysis) just before the attempt.

Factors that influence the success of an attempted version include multiparity, a posterior placenta, and normal amniotic fluid with a normally grown fetus. In addition, to be a candidate, a patient must be eligible for an attempted vaginal delivery.

Contraindications to external cephalic version inlclude oligohydramnios, intrauterine growth restriction with abnormal doppler or fetal heart tracing, major uterine anomalies, antepartum hemorrhage, abnormal fetal heart tracing, multiparity and rupture of memebrane.

Relative contraindications include poor fetal growth or the presence of congenital anomalies.

Risks of an external cephalic version include rupture of membranes, labor, fetal injury, and the need for an emergent CS due to placental abruption.

If the version is successful, the patient is placed on a fetal monitor in close proximity to the labor and delivery unit or in the labor and delivery unit itself.

If fetal heart rate testing is reassuring, the patient is discharged to await spontaneous labor, or she may be induced if the fetus is of an appropriate gestational age or the patient has a favorable cervix.

The first twin in a nonvertex presentation is an indication for a CS, as are higher order multiples (triplets or greater).

A large body of literature supports both outright CS as well as spontaneous breech delivery or extraction of the second twin.

The decision is made in conjunction with the patient after appropriate counseling regarding the risks and benefits as well as under the supervision of a physician experienced in the management of the labor and delivery of a breech fetus.

Evidence suggests that the rate of severe complications of the second breech twin is independent of the mode of delivery.

Several congenital anomalies are controversial indications for CS; these include fetal neural tube defects (to avoid sac rupture), particularly defects that are larger than 5-6 cm in diameter.

One study noted no difference in long-term neurologic outcomes.

Some authors noted no relationship between mode of delivery and infant outcomes, while others have advocated CS of all infants with a neural tube defect.

CS is indicated in certain cases of hydrocephalus with an enlarged biparietal diameter, and some skeletal dysplasias such as type III osteogenesis imperfecta.

Whether or not an outright CS should be performed in the setting of a fetal abdominal wall defect (eg, gastroschisis or omphalocele) remains controversial.

Most reviews agree that CS is not advantageous unless the liver is extruded, which is a very rare event.

The overall incidence of CS in this group of patients is probably due to an increased incidence of intrauterine growth retardation and fetal distress prior to or in labor.

In the setting of a nonremediable and nonreassuring pattern remote from delivery, a CS is recommended to prevent a mixed or metabolic acidemia that could potentially cause significant morbidity and mortality.

Electronic fetal monitoring was used in 85% of labors in the US in 2002.

Its use has increased the CS rate as much as 40%.

This has occurred without a decrease in the cerebral palsy or perinatal death rate.

ACOG has recommended that any facility providing obstetric care have the capability of performing a CS within 30 minutes of the decision.

Despite this recommendation, a decision to delivery time of more than 30 minutes is not necessarily associated with a negative neonatal outcome.

Among patients with culture-positive herpes, the transmission rate with vaginal delivery was 7 times that with CS.

Currently, all patients with active or symptomatic herpes infection are candidates for CS.

Neonatal infection with herpes can lead to significant morbidity and mortality, especially with a primary outbreak.

Unfortunately, not all women with active viral shedding can be detected upon admission to labor and delivery.

Treatment of women with HIV infections has undergone tremendous change in the past few years.

Women with a viral count above 1,000 should be offered CS at 38 weeks (or earlier if they go into labor).

In women who are being treated with highly active antiretroviral therapy (HAART), CS (before labor or without prolonged rupture of membranes) appears to further lower the risk for neonatal transmission, particularly among those with viral counts above 1,000.

Among patients with low or undetectable viral counts, the evidence supporting a benefit is not as clear; nevertheless, the patient should be given the option of a CS.

Breech

Transverse

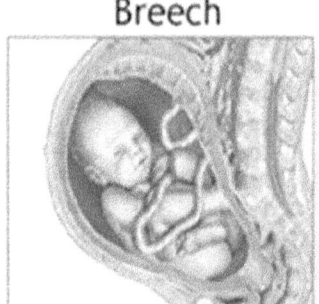 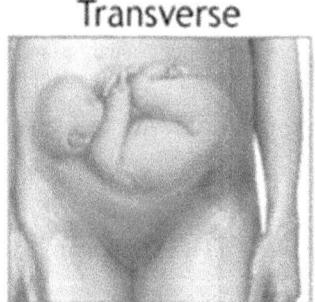

Malpresentations

MATERNAL/FETAL INDICATIONS

Indications for CS that benefit both the mother and the fetus include the following:

−Abnormal placentation.

−Abnormal labor due to cephalopelvic disproportion.

−Situations in which labor is contraindicated.

In the presence of a placenta previa (ie, the placenta covering the internal cervical os), attempting vaginal delivery places both the mother and the fetus at risk for hemorrhagic complications.

This complication has actually increased as a result of the increased incidence of repeat CS, which is a risk factor for placenta previa and placenta accreta.

Both placenta previa and placenta accreta carry increased morbidity related to hemorrhage and need for hysterectomy.

Cephalopelvic disproportion can be suspected on the basis of possible macrosomia or an arrest of labor despite augmentation.

Many cases diagnosed as cephalopelvic disproportion are the result of a primary or secondary arrest of dilatation or arrest of descent.

Predicting true primary or secondary arrest of descent due to cephalopelvic disproportion is best assessed by sagittal suture overlap, but not lambdoid suture overlap, particularly where progress is poor in a trial of labor.

Continuing to attempt a vaginal delivery in this setting increases the risk of infectious complications to both mother and fetus from prolonged rupture of membranes.

Less often, maternal hemorrhagic and fetal metabolic consequences occur from a uterine rupture, especially among patients with a previous CS.

Vaginal delivery can also increase the risk of maternal trauma and fetal trauma (eg, Erb-Duchenne or Klumpke palsy and metabolic acidosis) from a shoulder dystocia.

Among women who have a uterine scar (prior transmural myomectomy or CS by high vertical incision), a CS should be performed prior to the onset of labor to prevent the risk of uterine rupture, which is approximately 4-10%.

Placenta previa   Placenta abruptio

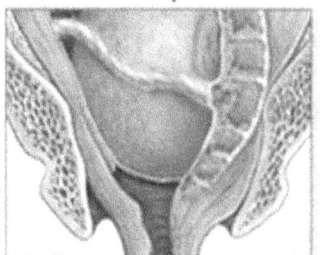 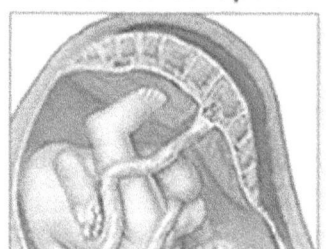

Abnormal Placentation

TECHNIQUE OF CS

The following are included in preoperative management:

– Timing of CS according to the indication.

– A minimum preoperative fasting time of at least 2 hours from clear liquids, 6 hours from a light meal, and 8 hours from a regular meal.

– Placement of an IV line.

– Infusion of IV fluids.

– Preoperative lab samples are drawn.

– Placement of an external fetal monitor and monitors for the patient's blood pressure, pulse, and oxygen saturation.

– Placement of a Foley catheter.

– Preoperative antibiotic prophylaxis.

– Evaluation by the surgeon and the anesthesiologist.

The technique for CS includes the following:

– Laparotomy via midline infraumbilical, vertical, or transverse (eg, Pfannenstiel, Mayland, Joel Cohen) incision.

– Hysterotomy via a transverse (Monroe-Kerr) or vertical (eg, Kronig, DeLee) incision.

– Fetal delivery.

−Uterine repair.

−Abdominal closure.

−If patient has been counseled and consented prior to the procedure, an IUD can be placed prior to the repair of the hysterotomy.

The following are included in postoperative management:

−Routine postoperative assessment.

−Monitoring of vital signs, urine output, and amount of vaginal bleeding.

−Palpation of the fundus.

−IV fluids; advance to oral diet as appropriate, early feeding has been shown to shorten hospital stay.

−IV or IM analgesia if patient did not receive a long-acting analgesic or had general anesthesia; analgesia is usually not needed if patient received regional anesthesia.

−Ambulation on postoperative day 1; advance as tolerated.

−If patient plans to breastfeed, initiate within a few hours after delivery; if patient plans to bottle feed, she may use a tight bra or breast binder in the postoperative period.

−Discharge on postoperative day 2 to 4, if no complications.

−Discuss contraception as well as refraining from intercourse for 4-6 weeks postpartum.

PREOPERATIVE MANAGEMENT

– Timing of CS according to the indication.

– The guidelines recommend a minimum preoperative fasting time of at least 2 hours from clear liquids, 6 hours from a light meal, and 8 hours from a regular meal.

– Placement of an IV line.

– Infusion of IV fluids (eg, lactated Ringer solution or saline with 5% dextrose).

– Preoperative lab samples are drawn.

– Placement of an external fetal monitor and monitors for the patient's blood pressure, pulse, and oxygen saturation.

– Placement of a Foley catheter (to drain the bladder and to monitor urine output).

– Preoperative antibiotic prophylaxis (decreases risk of endometritis after elective CS by 76%, regardless of the type of CS).

– Evaluation by the surgeon and the anesthesiologist.

– If a difficult procedure is anticipated with an increased risk for blood loss, cross-matched blood should be available for the start of the procedure.

Timing of CS

−Emergency CS:

Ideally the C.S should be done within the next 30 minutes.

Some examples are abruption, cord prolapse, scar rupture, scalp blood pH <7.20, and prolonged FHR deceleration.

−Urgent CS:

The delivery should be completed within 60-75 minutes.

Cases with FHR abnormalities are those of concern.

−Scheduled CS:

Continuation of pregnancy is likely to affect the mother or fetus in hours or days.

It may be a case of failure to progress where the CS is planed within next hours or it may be a case with preeclampsia where CS is planned for within hours to days.

−Elective CS:

The main principle is to carry out CS as late as possible in gestation without compromising the maternal or fetal health.

Examples include placenta previa or malpresentations.

Laboratory Investigations

When patients are admitted for labor and delivery, most have blood drawn for a complete blood count (CBC) and type and screen when an IV line is started, which is a basic requirement for patients when they are admitted to the labor floor.

If the patient has a hemoglobin level within the reference range, has had an uncomplicated pregnancy, and is anticipated to have a vaginal delivery, the utility of submitting blood to the lab for a routine CBC and type and screen has been debated from a cost-benefit standpoint.

In many centers, blood is drawn and simply held in case the patient's course changes.

If the decision is made to perform a CS for an abnormal labor course, nonreassuring fetal testing, or abnormal bleeding, then the blood work is submitted.

Several situations can occur in which a CBC count and type and screen will be submitted upon admission to labor and delivery:

– The patient is admitted for a planned CS.

– The patient is a grand multipara.

– The patient has a history of postpartum hemorrhage or a bleeding disorder.

In addition, tests for HIV antibodies and hepatitis B surface antigen and a screening test for syphilis are done, if these have not been recently obtained.

Occasionally, a coagulation profile is necessary.

In patients with thrombocytopenia, a history of a bleeding disorder, preeclampsia, or a condition with suspected disseminated intravascular coagulation (DIC), whether consumptive or secondary to thromboplastin release, a CBC and coagulation studies (including prothrombin time [PT], activated partial thromboplastin time [aPTT], and fibrinogen) may be ordered to assist the attending anesthesiologist in determining the safety of attempting regional anesthesia with an epidural or spinal procedure.

Most known thrombophilias, hemophilias, or other medical conditions that could compromise cardiac, circulatory, or respiratory function during surgery should be addressed with the anesthesiologist before admission for CS.

This includes patients with morbid obesity in which airway access as well as vascular access can be extremely challenging.

Some patients require blood to be cross-matched, with blood in storage available.

The most common situation is a patient who has had prior laparotomies (including CS), patients with known or suspect placenta previa or placenta accreta, or one who develops a coagulopathy from either severe preeclampsia or significant hemorrhage.

Preoperative Monitoring

A blood pressure cuff is placed; monitors are also placed to allow the blood pressure, pulse, and oxygen saturation to be monitored before administration of anesthesia through the initial postoperative period in the recovery room.

Before surgery, a Foley catheter is placed so that the bladder can be drained during the procedure and urine output can be monitored to help evaluate fluid status.

After regional anesthesia, patients are unable to void spontaneously for as long as 24 hours.

A review suggests that nonuse of indwelling urinary catheters in caesarean delivery is associated with fewer urinary tract infections and no increase in urinary retention or intraoperative difficulties.

Further trials are necessary to confirm this finding among patients who receive spinal or epidural anesthesia for uncomplicated CS.

Preoperative antibiotic prophylaxis decreases the risk of endometritis by 76%, regardless of the type of CS (emergent or elective).

There is evidence that IV prophylactic antibiotics for CS administered preoperatively significantly decrease the incidence of composite maternal postpartum infectious morbidity as compared with administration after cord clamp.

Further research may be required to elucidate short- and long-term adverse effects for neonates.

Single-dose therapy is recommended for its effectiveness, lower cost, decreased potential toxicity, and decreased development of resistance.

A first-generation cephalosporin is the first-line antibiotic of choice.

In women with penicillin or cephalosporin allergy (ie, anaphylaxis, angioedema, respiratory distress, or urticaria), the alternative is a combination of clindamycin with an aminoglycoside.

Adding azithromycin 500mg continuous IV to cefazolin about an hour prior to surgery further reduce risk of endometriosis and wound infection.

Prolonged surgery, excessive blood loss, and maternal obesity may require repeat or higher dosing.

A meta-analysis of three randomized trials supports the use of antibiotic prophylaxis for CS administered up to 60 minutes before skin incision rather than after umbilical cord clamping.

There is no benefit from oral antibiotics for eradication of methicillin-resistant Staphylococcus epidermidis (MRSA) colonization among patients in the health care setting, and oral antibiotics are not currently routinely recommended for the purpose of MRSA decolonization.

Routine screening of obstetric patients for MRSA colonization is not recommended.

For obstetric patients known to be MRSA colonized, a single dose of vancomycin can be added to the antibiotic prophylaxis regimen.

Vancomycin alone does not provide sufficient coverage for surgical prophylaxis.

Infective endocarditis prophylaxis is not recommended for vaginal delivery or CS.

Patients at highest potential risk for adverse cardiac outcomes who are undergoing vaginal delivery may benefit from prophylaxis.

Those at highest risk are women with cyanotic cardiac disease, recently repaired cyanotic heart disease, residual defects after repair, prosthetic valves, history of bacterial endocarditis, or history of heart transplant.

Mitral valve prolapse is not considered a lesion that ever needs infective endocarditis prophylaxis.

Upon arrival to labor and delivery, fetal position and estimated fetal weight should always be documented.

Ultrasonography is commonly used to estimate fetal weight despite evidence reporting the sensitivity of clinical and ultrasonographic prediction of macrosomia as 68% and 58%, respectively.

Despite the notion that estimations have an inherent margin of error, a physician's failure to assess fetal weight during pregnancy or labor constitutes a deviation from standards of practice.

Anesthesia

The anesthesiologist will review regional anesthetic techniques.

Regional anesthesia is used for 95% of planned CS in the US.

The 3 main regional anesthetic techniques are spinal, epidural, and combined spinal epidural.

Every patient is evaluated for general anesthesia in case an emergency should arise and establishment of an airway becomes necessary.

Patients undergoing local anesthesia were found to have a significantly lower difference between preoperative and postoperative hematocrit levels when compared with patients undergoing general anesthesia.

Women having either an epidural anesthesia or spinal have a lower estimated maternal blood loss.

After placement of the regional anesthetic, monitor the fetus until an adequate surgical level has been achieved.

When the level of anesthesia is adequate, the skin can be prepared either with an iodine scrub or with 4% chlorhexidine.

Before making the initial incision, grasp the patient's skin bilaterally with an instrument such as an Allis clamp at the level of and above the incision to confirm anesthesia up to the level of T4.

This ensures that the anesthetic level is appropriate.

The dermatomal level of anesthesia required for CS is higher than that required for labor analgesia.

A sensory block to the 10th thoracic dermatome is sufficient to achieve analgesia for labor, but for CS, the anesthetic level must be extended cephalad to at least the fourth thoracic dermatome to prevent nociceptive input from the peritoneal manipulation.

In patients who require a CS secondary to a problem arising during labor, the preparation follows essentially the same steps previously outlined.

The only major variation occurs if a patient requires general anesthesia prior to the procedure.

In that situation, before intubation, the patient should be prepped and draped and the surgical team should be ready to begin as soon as the patient's airway is secured.

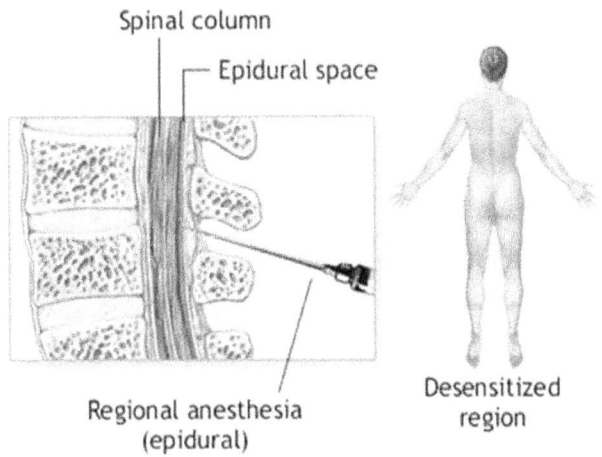

Epidural Anesthesia

OPERATIVE TECHNIQUE

As with any procedure, take care to avoid injury to adjacent organs.

Potential complications include bladder or bowel injury.

If a cystotomy or bowel injury is suspected, it should be evaluated thoroughly after the baby is delivered and hemostasis of the uterus is achieved.

The anesthesiologist monitors the patient's vital signs and tracks fluid intake and urine output.

The average blood loss associated with a CS is approximately 1000 mL.

A patient at term will have up to a 50% expansion in their blood volume and can lose up to 1500 mL without showing any change in vital signs.

If a significant blood loss is encountered or anticipated, assess the hemoglobin level and cross-match blood.

Most of the physiologic changes occurring during a CS are secondary to the physiologic adaptations to pregnancy, the medical or obstetrical complication affecting the mother, or secondary to obstetrical complications directly related to the pregnancy (eg, preeclampsia).

The method of anesthesia used also influences the physiologic adaptations that the mother undergoes during the procedure.

The use of chlorohexidine solution rather than a povidone iodine solution for sterilization is associated with a decrease risk of both superficial and deep wound infection.

Laparotomy

One option for entering the peritoneal cavity is to use a midline infraumbilical incision.

This incision provides quicker access to the uterus.

In pregnancy, entry is commonly enhanced by diastasis of the rectus muscles.

This incision is associated with less blood loss, easier examination of the upper abdomen, and easy extension cephalad around the umbilicus.

If there are likely to be significant intra-abdominal adhesions from previous operations, a vertical incision may provide easier access and better visualization.

Once the rectus sheath is reached, either the sheath can be incised with a scalpel for the entire length of the incision or a small incision in the fascia can be made with a scalpel and then extended superiorly and inferiorly with scissors.

Then, the rectus muscles (and pyramidalis muscles) are separated in the midline by sharp and blunt dissection.

This act exposes the transversalis fascia and the peritoneum.

The peritoneum is identified and entered at the superior aspect of the incision to avoid bladder injury.

Before entry into the peritoneum, care is taken to avoid incising adjacent bowel or omentum.

Once the peritoneal cavity is entered, the peritoneal incision is extended sharply to the upper aspect of the incision superiorly and to the reflection over the bladder inferiorly.

Most commonly, a transverse incision through lower abdomen is made.

The incision is a Maylard, Joel Cohen, or, more commonly, a Pfannenstiel incision.

Transverse incisions take slightly longer to enter the peritoneal cavity, are usually less painful, have been associated with a smaller risk of developing an incisional hernia, are preferred cosmetically, and can provide excellent visualization of the pelvis.

The Pfannenstiel incision is curved slightly cephalad at the level of the pubic hairline.

The incision extends slightly beyond the lateral borders of the rectus muscle bilaterally and is carried to the fascia.

Then, the fascia is incised bilaterally for the full length of the incision.

Then, the underlying rectus muscle is separated from the fascia both superiorly and inferiorly with blunt and sharp dissection.

Clamp and ligate any blood vessels encountered.

The rectus muscles are separated in the midline, and the peritoneum is entered.

A Maylard incision is made approximately 2-3 cm above the symphysis and is quicker than a Pfannenstiel incision.

It involves a transverse incision of the anterior rectus sheath and rectus muscle bilaterally.

Identify and possibly ligate the superficial inferior epigastric vessels (located in the lateral third of each rectus).

For CS, only the medial two thirds of each rectus muscle usually needs to be divided; if more than two thirds of the rectus muscle is divided, identify and ligate the deep inferior epigastric vessels.

The transversalis fascia and peritoneum are incised transversely.

The Joel Cohen incision is a straight transverse incision made 3 cm below the level of a straight line joining the anterosuperior iliac spines.

The skin incision is made and carried down to the anterior sheath of the rectus fascia.

A 3-4 cm incision is made in the fascia and bluntly opened by stretching in a craniocaudal fashion.

The rectus muscles are retracted laterally and the parietal peritoneum is bluntly opened by digital dissection.

The peritoneum is then retracted cephalocaudally to avoid injury to the bladder.

In comparison to the Pfannensteil incision, the Joel Cohen incision is associated with less blood loss, shorter operating time, reduced time to oral intake, less risk of fever, shorter duration of postoperative pain, lower analgesic requirements, and shorter time from skin incision to birth of the baby.

The Maylard incision with transection of the rectus muscles is associated with increased blood loss.

No evidence reports an advantage of electrocautery over sharp knife dissection or digital dissection of the subcutaneous tissues, or whether sharp or blunt retraction of the fascial tissues is preferable.

Blunt dissection tends to be associated with reduced blood loss.

Horizontal incision   Vertical incision

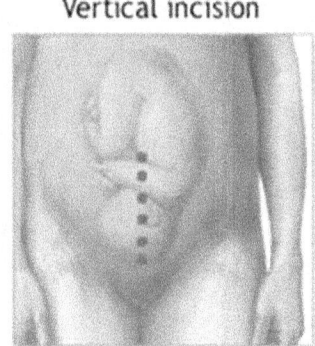

Laparotomy

Hysterotomy

Upon entering the peritoneal cavity by blunt or sharp dissection and blunt extension, inspect the lower abdomen.

The uterus is palpated and is commonly found to be dextrorotated, so that the left round ligament is more anterior and closer to the midline.

Evidence suggests that development of a bladder flap is not always necessary, especially in the nonlabored patient.

In creating a bladder flap, dissect the bladder free of the lower uterine segment.

Grasp the loose uterovesical peritoneum with forceps, and incise it with Metzenbaum scissors.

The incision is extended bilaterally in an upward curvilinear fashion.

The lower flap is grasped gently, and the bladder is separated from the lower uterus with blunt and sharp dissection.

A bladder blade is placed to both displace and protect the bladder inferiorly and to provide exposure for the lower uterine segment (the least contractile portion of the uterus).

Either a transverse (Monroe-Kerr) or a vertical (Kronig or DeLee) incision may be made on the uterus.

The choice of incision is based on several factors, including fetal presentation, gestational age, placental location, and presence of a well-developed lower uterine segment.

The incision selected must allow enough room to deliver the fetus without risking injury (either tearing or cutting) to the uterine arteries and veins that are located at the lateral margins of the uterus.

In more than 90% of CS, a low transverse (Monroe-Kerr) incision is made.

The incision is made 1-2 cm above the original upper margin of the bladder with a scalpel.

The initial incision is small and is continued into the uterine wall until either the fetal membranes are visualized or the cavity is entered

Care is taken to avoid injury the underlying fetus, especially in well-labored patients with thinned out lower uterine segments).

The incision is extended bilaterally and slightly cephalad.

The incision can be extended with either sharp dissection or blunt dissection (usually with the index fingers of the surgeon).

Blunt dissection is associated with decreased blood loss but has the potential for unpredictable extension, and care should be taken to avoid injury to the uterine vessels.

Uterine and vaginal extensions after a low transverse incision are more common after a prolonged second stage of labor and impaction of the fetal head.

The presenting part of the fetus is identified, and the fetus is delivered either as a vertex presentation or as a breech.

With a low transverse incision, the risk for uterine rupture in subsequent pregnancies is approximately 0.5-1%, and patients can be counseled about the safety of an attempted trial of labor and vaginal birth.

In some instances, a vertical incision is used.

Such incisions may be chosen if the lower segment is not well developed (ie, narrow), if an anterior placenta previa is present, or if the fetus is in a transverse lie or in a preterm nonvertex presentation.

Again, the bladder has been dissected inferiorly to expose the lower segment, and the bladder blade has been placed.

The vertical incision is initiated with a scalpel in the inferior portion of the lower uterine segment.

Care is taken to avoid injury to the underlying fetus, and the incision is carried into the uterus until the cavity is entered.

When the cavity is entered, the incision is extended superiorly with sharp dissection.

The fetus is identified and delivered.

Note the extent of the superior portion of the uterine incision.

If the incision is confined to the lower uterine segment, it is considered a low vertical incision, and patients can be counseled for a trial of labor and vaginal delivery in subsequent pregnancies.

With a true low vertical incision, the risk of uterine rupture with a trial of labor is similar to low transverse incision (less than 1.5%).

If the incision should be either extended into the contractile portion of the uterus or is made almost completely in the upper contractile portion, the risk of uterine rupture in future pregnancies is 4-10%, and patients are counseled to undergo a repeat CS with all subsequent pregnancies.

A vertical incision may also be considered when a hysterectomy may be planned in the setting of a placenta accreta or when the patient has a coexisting cervical cancer for which a hysterectomy would be the appropriate treatment.

A vertical incision is associated with a greater degree of blood loss and a longer operating time than a low transverse incision (because it takes longer to close) but poses less risk of injury to the uterine vessels.

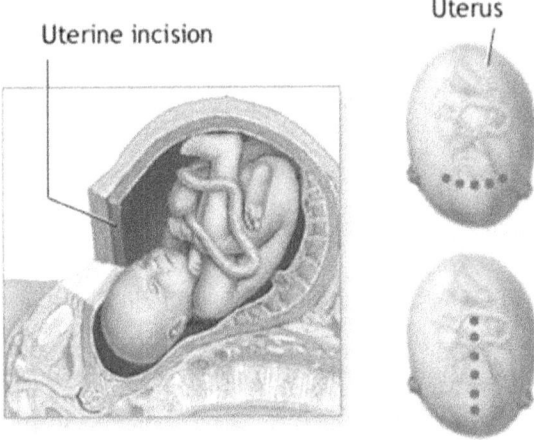

Hysterotomy

Fetal Delivery

Two important aspects of the delivery are (1) the incision to delivery time (especially in previously compromised fetuses) and (2) delivery of the impacted fetal head.

Longer incision to delivery time is associated with worsening neonatal outcomes.

The impacted fetal head can be delivered either through pushing the head up from the vagina and elevating it up through the incision or by pulling it up as if it were a breech delivery.

This may require extending the incision to make room to maneuver.

After the fetus is delivered, the umbilical cord is doubly clamped and cut.

Blood is obtained from the cord for fetal blood typing, and a segment of cord is placed aside for obtaining blood gas results if a concern exists regarding fetal status.

After delivery, oxytocin (20 U) is placed in the IV fluid to increase contractions of the uterus.

The placenta is usually delivered manually.

Awaiting spontaneous delivery of the placenta with gentle traction on the cord is more time consuming but is associated with decreased blood loss, lower risk of endometritis, and lower maternal exposure to fetal red blood cells, which can be important to Rh-negative mothers delivering an Rh-positive fetus.

If the surgery is prolonged, a second dose of antibiotic can be administered every 2 hours to maintain adequate serum concentrations.

If the patient has chorioamnionitis, broader-spectrum antibiotics, such as gentamicin and clindamycin or penicillin with a beta-lactamase inhibitor, are indicated and should be continued in the postoperative period until the patient is afebrile.

If MRSA is suspected as a pathogen, especially in abdominal wall infections, vancomycin will have to be added.

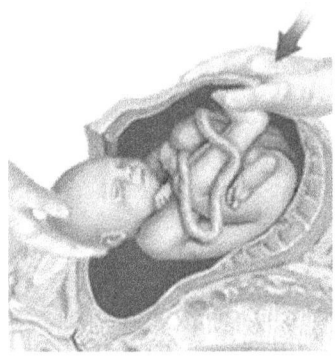 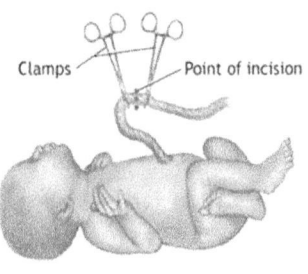

Fetal Delivery

Uterine Repair

Repair of the uterus can be facilitated by manual delivery of the uterine fundus through the abdominal incision.

Externalizing the uterine fundus facilitates uterine massage, the ability to assess whether the uterus is atonic, and the examination of the uterine incision and adnexa.

The uterine cavity is usually wiped clean of all membranes with a dry laparotomy sponge.

Typically, a clamp is placed at the angles of the uterine incision.

The incision is inspected for other bleeding vessels, and any extensions of the incision are evaluated. Inspect the bladder and lower segment inferior to the incision.

Repair of a low transverse uterine incision should be performed in either a 1-layer or 2-layer fashion with 0 or 2-0 chromic or polyglactin suture.

The first layer should include stitches placed lateral to each angle, with prior palpation of the location of the lateral uterine vessels.

Most physicians use a continuous locking stitch.

If the first layer is hemostatic, the second layer (Lembert stitch), which is used to imbricate the incision, need not be placed.

Although single-layer closure, compared with double-layer closure, was associated with a statistically significant reduction in mean blood loss, duration of the operative procedure, and presence of postoperative pain.

Recent studies have shown that 2-layer closures are associated with a significant decrease in the rate of uterine rupture in subsequent pregnancy and current ACOG recommendations support 2-layer closures in women who plan on having more children.

At least 1 study reported a 4-fold increase in the risk of uterine rupture when comparing 2- to 1-layer closure.

Closure of a vertical incision usually requires several layers because the incision was made through a thicker portion of the uterus.

Again, a heavy suture material is used, and usually the first layer closes the inner half of the incision, with a second and possibly a third layer used to close the outer half and serosal edges.

The extent of a vertical uterine incision influences how a patient should be counseled regarding future pregnancies.

Once the uterus has been closed, attention must be paid to its overall tone.

An atonic uterus can be encountered in a patient with a multiple gestation, polyhydramnios, or a failed attempt at a vaginal delivery in which the patient was on oxytocin augmentation for a prolonged period.

If the uterus does not feel firm and contracted with massage and IV oxytocin, consider IM injections of prostaglandin or methyl-ergonovine, and repeat as appropriate.

If the patient has been consented prior to her CS for an intrauterine device (IUD) the device is placed prior to closing the uterine incision.

The device is placed at the fundus with the strings toward the cervical os.

The strings should not be placed into the vagina from above, evidence shows that the strings will migrate in the direction of the cervical canal and into the vagina.

Immediate postpartum insertion of an IUD after a CS is associated with a lower expulsion rate than after a vaginal delivery.

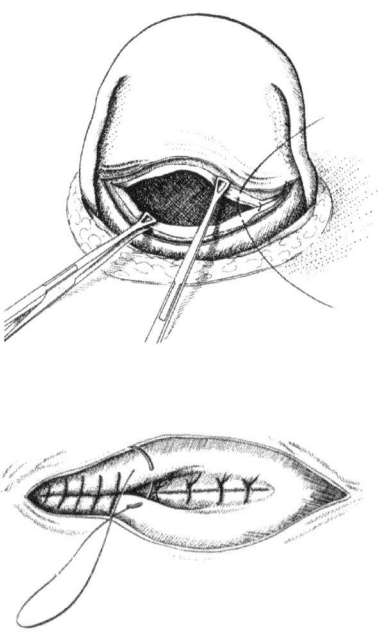

Uterine Repair

Abdominal Closure

If the uterine incision is hemostatic, the uterine fundus is replaced into the abdominal cavity (unless a concurrent tubal ligation is to be performed).

The incision is re-inspected for hemostasis, and the bladder flap is also inspected.

The paracolic gutters are visualized, and any blood clots are removed with laparotomy sponges.

Although many surgeons perform abdominal irrigation, this does not appear advantageous.

Peritoneal closure is no longer recommended as it is associated with increased adhesion formation and may increase surgical time as well as length of hospital stay.

Furthermore these surfaces reapproximate within 24-48 hours and can heal without scar formation.

Furthermore, the rectus muscles to do not need to be reapproximated.

The subfascial and muscle tissue is inspected for bleeding, and, if hemostatic, the fascia is closed.

The fascia can be closed with a running nonlocking stitch, and synthetic braided or monofilament sutures are preferred over chromic sutures.

Chromic sutures do not maintain their tensile strength as long or as predictably as synthetic material.

If the patient is at risk for poor wound healing (eg, from long-term steroid use), a delayed absorbable or permanent suture can be used.

Place stitches at approximately 1-cm intervals and more than 1 cm away from the incision line.

The subcutaneous tissue should be inspected for hemostasis and can be irrigated according to physician preference.

The subcutaneous tissue usually does not have to be reapproximated, but patients with subcutaneous depth greater than 2 cm may benefit from subcutaneous tissue closure.

Placement of drains is no longer recommended and has been shown to increase the risk of infection.

If needed, a closed vacuum suction system should be used in the appropriate patients.

The skin edges should be closed with a subcuticular stitch as staples have shown to be associated with increased wound infection and wound disruption.

If the patient has consented to a levonorgestrel subdermal implant prior to her CS, then the device should be inserted in the patient's non-dominant arm using standard procedure.

POSTOPERATIVE MANAGEMENT

−Routine postoperative assessment.

−Monitoring of vital signs, urine output, and amount of vaginal bleeding.

−Palpation of the fundus.

−IV fluids; advance to oral diet as appropriate, early feeding has been shown to shorten hospital stay.

−IV or IM analgesia if patient did not receive a long-acting analgesic or had general anesthesia; analgesia is usually not needed if patient received regional anesthesia, with/without a long-acting analgesic.

−Ambulation on postoperative day 1; advance as tolerated.

−If patient plans to breastfeed, initiate within a few hours after delivery; if patient plans to bottle feed, she may use a tight bra or breast binder in the postoperative period.

−Discharge on postoperative day 2 to 4, if no complications.

−Discuss contraception as well as refraining from intercourse for 4-6 weeks postpartum, unless the patient had LARC placed at the time of the procedure.

Postoperative Care

In the recovery room, vital signs are taken every 15 minutes for the first 1-2 hours, and urine output is monitored on an hourly basis.

Palpate the fundus to ensure that it feels firm; pay attention to the amount of vaginal bleeding.

If the patient had regional anesthesia, they usually receive a long-acting analgesic with the regional anesthetic; therefore, pain control is usually not an issue in the first 24 hours.

If a patient did not receive a long-acting analgesic or had general anesthesia, administer narcotics either IM or IV, on schedule or with a basal rate supplemented with patient-controlled boluses.

When the patient is tolerating liquids, administer narcotics orally.

Vital signs should be taken every hour for at least the first 4 hours - again, with particular attention paid to urine output.

Overall, a patient should receive approximately 3-4 L of IV fluid from the initiation of IV fluid replacement through the first 24 hours.

The patient can be started on clear liquids 12-24 hours after an uncomplicated procedure, and diet can be advanced accordingly.

When the patient is able to tolerate good oral intake, the IV fluids may be stopped.

The bladder catheter can be removed 12-24 hours postoperatively once the patient is ambulatory.

On the first postoperative day, encourage the patient to ambulate.

The dressing can be removed 12-24 hours after surgery and can be left open after that time.

Typically, the blood count is checked 12-24 hours after surgery, or sooner if a greater than average blood loss has occurred.

If a patient plans to breastfeed, this can be initiated within a few hours after delivery.

If a patient plans to bottle feed, a tight bra or breast binder should be used in the postoperative period.

If the patient has recovered well postoperatively, she can be discharged safely 2-4 days after surgery.

Before discharge, a discussion about contraception should take place unless the patient had immediate postpartum LARC placement.

Stress that even if a mother is breastfeeding, she still can conceive.

Ask patients to refrain from intercourse for 4-6 weeks postpartum.

Long-Term Monitoring

After a CS, the patient can be observed as a patient who delivered vaginally.

The normal recommendation is to have the patient make a follow-up appointment 4-6 weeks after delivery.

During this visit, review any notable findings from the surgery and discuss delivery options for future pregnancies.

If bleeding has stopped, a repeat Papanicolaou test as needed based on recent pap screening guidelines is customary.

1 day after   1 year after

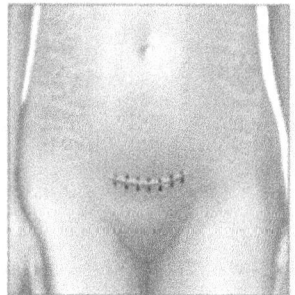 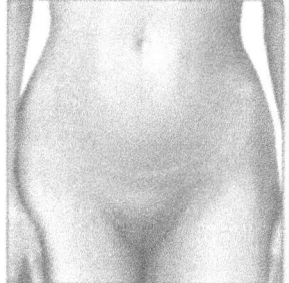

CS Scar

Expected Outcomes

Patients who undergo CS usually take slightly longer to fully recover than those who have a vaginal delivery.

Occasionally, some patients can experience pelvic pain associated with intra-abdominal adhesions, a situation that can be aggravated in those who have multiple procedures.

The most important things for patients to know about their CS are why they had one and what kind of incision was performed on the uterus.

If a patient had a CS for presumed cephalopelvic disproportion, then attempting a vaginal birth with the next pregnancy is associated with a decreased chance of success.

If the CS was performed because of an abnormal fetal heart pattern or for a malpresentation, then expectations for a successful vaginal birth can be higher than 70%.

If the uterine incision was vertical, the risk of uterine rupture is increased above the approximate 1% risk associated with a low transverse incision.

If the incision was confined to the lower segment, many physicians allow patients to attempt a vaginal birth in subsequent pregnancies.

A previous CS can increase the risk of developing placenta accreta if placenta previa is present in any subsequent pregnancies.

COMPLICATIONS OF CS

Compared with a vaginal delivery, maternal mortality and especially morbidity is increased with CS to approximately twice the rate after a vaginal delivery.

The overall maternal mortality rate is 6-22 deaths per 100,000 live births, with approximately one third to one half of maternal deaths after CS being directly attributable to the operative procedure itself.

Part of this increase in mortality is that associated with a surgical procedure and, in part, related to the conditions that may have led to needing to perform a CS.

Major sources of morbidity and mortality can be related to sequelae of surgical injury, anesthetic complications, infection, and thromboembolic disease.

One study indicated that despite clinical pressure to delay delivery until 39 weeks' gestation, waiting to reach this benchmark before performing a repeat CS may increase maternal risk.

According to the study, optimal time of delivery is 38 weeks for women with 2 previous CS and 37 weeks for those with 3 or more.

The investigation involved 6435 women who had delivered a singleton weighing more than 500 g at a gestational age of at least 20 weeks.

All women had undergone at least 2 previous low transverse CS and had plans for a repeat procedure; all delivered at 37 weeks or later.

For women with 2 previous CS, the risk for adverse maternal outcomes was 3.3 per 1000 women undelivered.

As gestational age at delivery increased, so did this risk, which approached 15.0 per 1000 for delivery at 39 weeks.

For women with 3 or more previous CS, the risk for adverse maternal outcome rose from less than 5.0 per 1000 deliveries at week 37 to 30.0 at week 39 and to 50.0 at week 40.

However, this must be balanced with recent findings that infants delivered between 37 and 38 weeks and 6 days have higher morbidity and mortality then infants delivered after 39 weeks.

In 2013, ACOG and Society for Maternal-Fetal Medicine (SMFM) made the joint recommendation to reconsider the old gestational age classification given those findings and replaced them with the following definitions of gestational age:

–Early term (37 0/7 weeks to 38 6/7 weeks).

–Full term (39 0/7 weeks to 40 6/7 weeks).

–Late term (41 0/7 weeks to 41 6/7 weeks).

–Post term (42 weeks and above).

OPERATIVE COMPLICATIONS

Uterine lacerations, especially of the lower uterine segment, are more common with a transverse uterine incision.

These lacerations can extend laterally or inferiorly; they are easily repaired.

Take care to identify the uterine vessels when repairing lateral extensions, and think about the ureters when repairing inferior extensions.

If the laceration extends into the broad ligament, strongly consider opening the broad ligament medial to the ovaries and identifying the course of the ureters.

Bladder injury is an infrequent complication; it is more common with transverse abdominal incisions and in repeat CS.

The bladder most commonly is injured during entry into the peritoneal cavity or when the bladder is separated from the lower uterine segment.

Bladder injury has been reported to occur in more than 10% of uterine ruptures and in approximately 4% of cesarean hysterectomies.

If a possibility exists that a cesarean hysterectomy may be performed, mobilize the bladder inferiorly as well as possible when dissecting it free of the lower uterine segment.

If the dome of the bladder is lacerated, it can be repaired simply with a 2-layer closure of 2-0 or 3-0 chromic sutures, with the Foley catheter left in place for a few extra days.

If the bladder is injured in the region of the trigone, consider ureteral catheterization with possible assistance from a urologist.

Injury to the ureter occurs in up to 0.1% of all CS and up to 0.5% of cesarean hysterectomies.

It is most likely to occur in the repair of extensive lacerations of the uterus.

Ureteral injury, most commonly occlusion or transection, is usually not recognized during the time of the operation.

Bowel injuries occur in less than 0.1% of all CS.

The most common risk factor for bowel injury at the time of CS is adhesions from prior CS or prior bowel surgery.

Injuries to the serosa can be repaired with interrupted silk sutures.

If the injury is into the lumen, perform a 2-layer closure.

For multiple injuries and injury to the large intestine, consider intraoperative consultation with a general surgeon.

Uterine atony is another intraoperative complication that can be encountered in a patient with a multiple gestation, polyhydramnios, or a failed attempt at a vaginal delivery in which the patient was on oxytocin augmentation for a prolonged period.

POSTOPERATIVE COMPLICATIONS

Postpartum endomyometritis is increased significantly in patients who have had a CS.

The rate of endomyometritis is up to 20-fold higher than with a vaginal delivery.

The postcesarean rate of endomyometritis can be decreased to approximately 5% with the use prophylactic antibiotics.

Major risk factors for endomyometritis include whether the CS was the intended (primary) procedure and the socioeconomic status of the patient.

Other major risk factors include duration of membrane rupture, duration of labor, number of pelvic examinations, length of time with internal fetal monitors in place, and presence of chorioamnionitis prior to initiating CS.

Blood cultures are positive in 10% of patients with postoperative febrile morbidity, and broad-spectrum antibiotics should be used.

After a CS, the risk of a wound infection ranges from 2.5% to 15%.

Risk factors are similar to those noted for endomyometritis, with the lowest risk associated with those having a planned CS.

If chorioamnionitis is present at the time of the procedure, the risk for a wound infection can be as high as 20%.

If a wound infection is suspected, open, irrigate, and débride the incision.

Then, the open wound can be packed and cleaned several times a day.

The wound can be allowed to heal by secondary intention, or, when it has begun to granulate, it can be closed.

With regard to vacuum-assisted closure in obese gravidas with wound disruption, level III evidence suggests that vacuum therapy can be included as an option for management of abdominal wounds, but evidence from randomized controlled trials in obese women undergoing CS is not available.

Research regarding the management of disrupted laparotomy wounds; overall, seems to support primary over delayed closure unless the wound is contaminated.

Infected wounds should be opened and drained and antibiotic therapy should be added if cellulitis or systemic toxicity is present.

Fascial dehiscence is an infrequent complication of a wound breakdown but constitutes a surgical emergency when it occurs.

It develops in approximately 5% of patients with a wound infection and is suggested when excessive discharge from the wound is present.

If a fascial dehiscence is observed, the patient should be taken immediately to the operating room, where the wound can be opened, débrided, and reclosed in a sterile environment.

The second most common etiology for postcesarean febrile morbidity is urinary tract infection (UTI).

The incidence ranges from 2-16%, and the process of placing an indwelling catheter for the surgery is a risk factor in itself.

The incidence of UTIs is increased in patients with diabetes, those who have other comorbidities, and those who have a longer duration of use of the indwelling catheter.

Postoperatively, some patients may experience a slow return of bowel function.

Postoperative narcotics may delay return of normal bowel function in a few patients.

Most respond to conservative therapy, but a small portion may require decompression.

In those with a slow return of bowel function, assessment of fluid and electrolyte status must be a priority.

Thromboembolic complications are also increased in patients who have undergone a CS.

Approximately 0.5-1 in 500 pregnant women experience deep venous thrombosis (DVT).

The risk for developing a thrombus is increased 3- to 5-fold with a CS and in the postpartum period.

Other risks include obesity, advanced maternal age, higher parity, and poor postoperative ambulation.

In those with risk factors for thromboembolism, consider pneumatic compression stockings or, in patients with additional risk factors, low-molecular-weight heparin.

If DVT is not treated, up to one quarter of patients will develop pulmonary emboli and 15% of these could be fatal. DVT is sometimes difficult to diagnose, and the first sign may be a pulmonary embolus.

Another infection-related complication of a CS is septic pelvic thrombophlebitis.

As many as 2% of patients with an endomyometritis or wound infection can develop this complication, and it is largely a diagnosis of exclusion.

Suspect this diagnosis if a patient fails to respond initially to broad-spectrum antibiotics.

Physical examination may detect a tender cordlike mass lateral to the uterus.

Ultrasonography, pelvic computed tomography (CT) scanning, or magnetic resonance imaging (MRI) may aid in the diagnosis.

Some authors advocate placing patients on therapeutic heparin along with continuing broad-spectrum antibiotics.

The length of adequate treatment once a patient has defervesced is subject to debate (anywhere from 48-h afebrile to a total of 7-10 d of treatment).

After completing the desired treatment course, patients do not need to be anticoagulated further.

HOW TO REDUCE CS RATE?

Decreasing the rate of primary CS and increased implementation of VBAC are important steps of a larger movement towards decreasing the overall rate of CS.

Recently ACOG and SMFM issued joint guidelines providing a framework for individual organizations and key players at the state and federal level to work with local hospitals to set the agenda to decrease the rate of primary CS.

Decreasing the rate of primary CS will result in a decreased number of repeat CS.

A large prospective randomized study is needed to look at single-layer versus double-layer closure and risk of future uterine rupture when a trial of labor is attempted after previous low-transverse CS.

The recommendation that all breech presentations should be delivered by a CS is currently a subject of active debate.

Additional information is required to address this issue in the setting of appropriately trained physicians and under well-established guidelines.

Urogynecologists suggest that all women should consider outright CS to prevent pelvic floor dysfunction.

This is an extremely controversial area that continues to receive attention, particularly in that short-term outcomes do not appear to relate to long-term outcomes.

PREVENTION OF PRIMARY CS

In 2014, 32.2% of women who gave birth in the US did so by CS.

The rapid increase in CS birth rates from 1996 to 2014 without clear evidence of concomitant decreases in maternal or neonatal morbidity or mortality raises significant concern that CS is overused.

The most common indications for primary CS include labor dystocia, abnormal or indeterminate fetal heart rate tracing, fetal malpresentation, multiple gestation, and suspected fetal macrosomia.

Safe reduction of the primary CS rate will require different approaches for these indications, as well as others.

Increasing women's access to nonmedical interventions during labor has also been shown to reduce CS birth rates.

The effects of continuous support on CS appeared to be stronger in settings which did not permit the presence of additional support people and when epidural was not routinely available.

External cephalic version for breech presentation and a trial of labor for women with twin gestations when the first twin is in cephalic presentation are examples of interventions that can help to safely lower the primary CS rate.

A practice bulletin from the ACOG recommends that all eligible women with breech presentations who are near term should be offered external cephalic version to decrease the overall rate of CS.

The ACOG and the SMFM released joint guidelines for the safe prevention of primary CS:

–Prolonged latent (early)-phase labor should be permitted.

–The start of active-phase labor can be defined as cervical dilation of 6 cm, rather than 4 cm.

–In the active phase, more time should be permitted for labor to progress.

–Multiparous women should be allowed to push for 2 or more hours and primiparous women for 3 or more hours; pushing may be allowed to continue for even longer periods in some cases, as when epidural anesthesia is administered.

–Techniques to aid vaginal delivery, such as the use of forceps, should be employed.

–Patients should be encouraged to avoid excessive weight gain during pregnancy.

–Access to nonmedical interventions during labor, such as continuous support during labor and delivery, should be increased.

–External cephalic version should be performed for breech presentation.

–Women with twin gestations should, if the first twin is in cephalic presentation, be permitted a trial of labor.

VAGINAL BIRTH AFTER CS (VBAC)

One of the most common dictums in obstetrics was put by Edward Craigin "Once a cesarean, always a cesarean".

From 1916, when these words were spoken to the New York Association of Obstetricians & Gynecologists, through the ensuing 50-60 years, this statement reflected most of US obstetricians' management of prior CS.

By 1988, the overall CS rate was 25%, rising from 5% in the early 1970s.

Although attempts at a trial of labor after a CS (TOLAC) have become accepted practice, the rate of successful VBACs, as well as the rate of attempted VBACs, has decreased during the past years.

Nevertheless, despite the known risks (0.5-1% rate of uterine rupture), TOLAC remains an attractive option for many patients and leads to a successful outcome in a high proportion of cases.

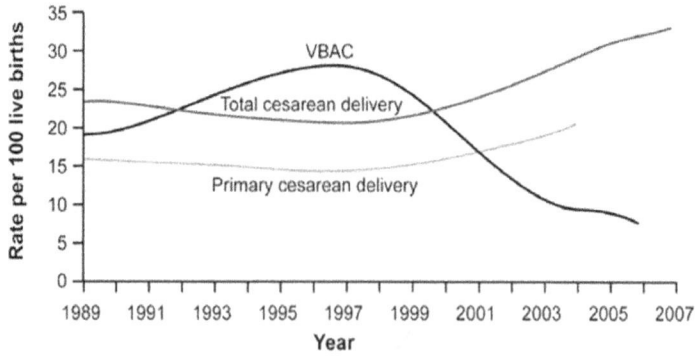

Rates of VBAC in US

ACOG Guidelines

On the basis of level A evidence, the 2010 ACOG guidelines make the following recommendations:

– Most women with a prior CS with a low transverse incision are candidates for VBAC and should be offered TOLAC.

– Epidural anesthesia may be used as part of TOLAC.

– Misoprostol should not be used for patients who have had a prior CS or major uterine surgery.

On the basis of level B evidence, TOLAC may be considered for the following patients:

– Women with 2 previous low transverse CS.

– Women with 1 previous CS with a low transverse incision who are otherwise appropriate candidates for twin vaginal delivery.

– Women with 1 previous CS of unknown incision type, unless clinical suspicion of a previous classical uterine incision is high.

Level B evidence was also found for the following:

– Induction of labor during TOLAC is not contraindicated.

– In women with a prior low transverse uterine incision who are at low risk for adverse maternal or neonatal outcomes from external cephalic version and TOLAC, external cephalic version for breech presentation is not contraindicated.

Technique of TOLAC

Patients with prior CS require special management, both antenatally and in labor and delivery.

Early in their prenatal care, catalogue patient's preexisting risk factors for both successful VBAC and uterine rupture.

Counsel the patient regarding the risks and benefits of undergoing a TOLAC.

Regarding management on labor and delivery, several practices can help to minimize the maternal and neonatal risk.

Have an obstetrician, anesthesiologist, and operating room team immediately available to carry out an emergency delivery.

Harbingers of uterine rupture include the following:

−Acute abdominal pain, persistent beyond contractions.

−A popping sensation.

−Palpation of fetal parts outside the uterus upon Leopold maneuvers.

−Repetitive or prolonged fetal heart rate deceleration.

−High presenting part upon vaginal examination.

−Vaginal bleeding.

Treat any of these findings as a possible uterine rupture until another finding has been identified; rupture necessitates immediate delivery.

Outcomes of TOLAC

Two specific outcomes regarding TOLAC have been well investigated:

(1) Predictors of VBAC Success

Increased chance of success:

- Prior vaginal delivery.

- Prior VBAC.

- Spontaneous labor.

- Favorable cervix.

- Nonrecurring indication (breech presentation, placenta previa, herpes).

- Preterm delivery.

Decreased chance of success:

- Maternal obesity.

- Short maternal stature.

- Macrosomia.

- Increased maternal age (>40 y).

- Induction of labor.

- Recurring indication (cephalopelvic disproportion, failed second stage).

- Increased interpregnancy weight gain.

− Latina or African American race/ethnicity.

− Gestational age ≥41 weeks.

− Preconceptional or gestational diabetes mellitus.

(2) Predictors of Uterine Rupture

Increased rate of uterine rupture:

− Classic hysterotomy.

− Two or more CSs.

− Single-layer closure.

− Induction of labor.

− Use of prostaglandins.

− Short interpregnancy interval.

− Infection at prior CS.

Decreased rate of uterine rupture:

− Spontaneous labor.

− Prior vaginal delivery.

− Longer interpregnancy interval.

− Preterm delivery.

REFERENCES

– ACOG Committee Opinion No. 340: Mode of term singleton breech delivery. *Obstet Gynecol.* 2006; 108(1): 235-7.

– ACOG Committee Opinion No. 579: Definition of term pregnancy. *Obstet Gynecol.* 2013; 122(5): 1139-40.

– ACOG Committee Opinion No. 670: Immediate postpartum long-acting reversible contraception. *Obstet Gynecol.* 2016; 128(2): 422-3.

– ACOG Practice Bulletin No. 49: Dystocia and augmentation of labor. *Obstet Gynecol.* 2003; 102(6): 1445-54.

– ACOG Practice Bulletin No. 115: Vaginal birth after previous cesarean delivery. *American College of Obstetricians and Gynecologists (ACOG).* Washington (DC): American College of Obstetricians and Gynecologists (ACOG); 2010.

– ACOG Practice Bulletin No. 120: Use of prophylactic antibiotics in labor and delivery. *Obstet Gynecol.* 2011; 117(6): 1472-83.

– Afolabi B, Lesi F, Merah N. Regional versus general anaesthesia for caesarean section. *Cochrane Database Syst Rev.* 2006; CD004350.

– Alexander J, Leveno K, Rouse D, et al. Cesarean delivery for the second twin. *Obstet Gynecol.* 2008; 112(4): 748-52.

– American College of Obstetricians and Gynecologists, Society for Maternal-Fetal Medicine. Obstetric care consensus No. 1: safe prevention of the primary cesarean delivery. *Obstet Gynecol.* 2014; 123(3): 693-711.

– Basha S, Rochon M, Quiñones J, et al. Randomized controlled trial of wound complication rates of subcuticular suture vs staples for skin closure at cesarean delivery. *Am J Obstet Gynecol.* 2010; 203(3): 285.e1-8.

– Berghella V, Baxter J, Chauhan S. Evidence-based surgery for cesarean delivery. *Am J Obstet Gynecol.* 2005; 193(5): 1607-17.

– Betran A, Merialdi M, Lauer J, et al. Rates of caesarean section: analysis of global, regional and national estimates. *Paediatr Perinat Epidemiol.* 2007; 21(2): 98-113.

– Brown H, Hiett A. Deep vein thrombosis and pulmonary embolism in pregnancy: diagnosis, complications, and management. *Clin Obstet Gynecol.* 2010; 53(2): 345-59.

– Brown Z, Wald A, Morrow R, et al. Effect of serologic status and cesarean delivery on transmission rates of herpes simplex virus from mother to infant. *JAMA.* 2003; 289(2): 203-9.

– Buchmann J, Libhaber E. Sagittal suture overlap in cephalopelvic disproportion: blinded and non-participant assessment. *Acta Obstet Gynecol Scand.* 2008; 87(7): 731-7.

– Bucklin B, Hawkins J, Anderson J, et al. Obstetric anesthesia workforce survey: twenty-year update. *Anesthesiology.* 2005; 103(3): 645-53.

– Bujold E, Bujold C, Hamilton E, et al. The impact of a single-layer or double-layer closure on uterine rupture. *Am J Obstet Gynecol.* 2002; 186(6): 1326-30.

– Bujold E, Gauthier R. Risk of uterine rupture associated with an interdelivery interval between 18 and 24 months. *Obstet Gynecol.* 2010; 115(5): 1003-6.

– Bujold E, Goyet M, Marcoux S, et al. The role of uterine closure in the risk of uterine rupture. *Obstet Gynecol.* 2010; 116(1):43-50.

– Caughey A, Cahill A, Guise J, et al. Safe prevention of the primary cesarean delivery. *Am J Obstet Gynecol.* 2014; 210(3): 179-93.

– Chaillet N, Dumont A, Abrahamowicz M, et al. A cluster-randomized trial to reduce cesarean delivery rates in Quebec. *N Engl J Med.* 2015; 372(18): 1710-21.

– Chelmow D, Rodriguez E, Sabatini M. Suture closure of subcutaneous fat and wound disruption after cesarean delivery: a meta-analysis. *Obstet Gynecol.* 2004; 103(5 Pt 1): 974-80.

– Cheng Y, Hopkins L, Laros R, et al. Duration of the second stage of labor in multiparous women: maternal and neonatal outcomes. *Am J Obstet Gynecol.* 2007; 196(6): 585.e1-6.

– Cho M, Kim Y, Song T. Predictive factors for vaginal birth after cesarean delivery. *Int J Gynaecol Obstet.* 2004; 86(3): 392-3.

– Chopra S, Bagga R, Keepanasseril A, et al. Disengagement of the deeply engaged fetal head during cesarean section in advanced labor: conventional method versus reverse breech extraction. *Acta Obstet Gynecol Scand.* 2009; 88(10): 1163-6.

– Chu S, Kim S, Schmid C, et al. Maternal obesity and risk of cesarean delivery: a meta-analysis. *Obes Rev.* 2007; 8(5): 385-94.

– Coleman-Cowger V, Erickson K, Spong C, et al. Current practice of cesarean delivery on maternal request following the 2006 state-of-the-science conference. *J Reprod Med.* 2010; 55(1-2): 25-30.

– Consortium on Safe Labor, Hibbard J, Wilkins I, Sun L, et al. Respiratory morbidity in late preterm births. *JAMA.* 2010; 304(4): 419-25.

– Costantine M, Rahman M, Ghulmiyah L, et al. Timing of perioperative antibiotics for cesarean delivery: a metaanalysis. *Am J Obstet Gynecol.* 2008; 199(3): 301.e1-6.

– Coutinho I, Ramos de Amorim M, Katz L, et al. Uterine exteriorization compared with in situ repair at cesarean delivery: a randomized controlled trial. *Obstet Gynecol.* 2008; 111(3): 639-47.

– Crenshaw J, Winslow E. Actual versus instructed fasting times and associated discomforts in women having scheduled cesarean birth. *J Obstet Gynecol Neonatal Nurs.* 2006; 35(2): 257-64.

– Cruikshank D. Intrapartum management of twin gestations. *Obstet Gynecol.* 2007; 109(5): 1167-76.

– Cunningham F, Bangdiwala S, Brown S, et al. NIH consensus development conference draft statement on vaginal birth after cesarean: new insights. *NIH Consens State Sci Statements.* 2010; 27(3): 1-42.

– Cunningham F, FLeveno K, Bloom S, et al. *Williams Obstetrics.* 23rd ed. Norwalk, Conn: Appleton & Lange; 2009.

– Dahlke J, Mendez H, Rouse D, et al. Evidence-based surgery for cesarean delivery: an updated systematic review. *Am J Obstet Gynecol.* 2013; 209(4): 294-306.

– Darney B, Snowden J, Cheng Y, et al. Elective induction of labor at term compared with expectant management: maternal and neonatal outcomes. *Obstet Gynecol.* 2013; 122(4): 761-9.

– Darouiche R, Wall M, Itani K, et al. Chlorhexidine-Alcohol versus Povidone-Iodine for Surgical-Site Antisepsis. *N Engl J Med.* 2010; 362(1): 18-26.

– Dodd J, Anderson E, Gates S. Surgical techniques for uterine incision and uterine closure at the time of caesarean section. *Cochrane Database Syst Rev.* 2008; CD004732.

– Durnwald C, Mercer B. Uterine rupture, perioperative and perinatal morbidity after single-layer and double-layer closure at cesarean delivery. *Am J Obstet Gynecol.* 2003; 189(4): 925-9.

– Faiz A, Ananth C. Etiology and risk factors for placenta previa: an overview and meta-analysis of observational studies. *J Matern Fetal Neonatal Med.* 2003; 13(3): 175-90.

– Foley M, Alarab M, Daly L, et al. Term neonatal asphyxial seizures and peripartum deaths: lack of correlation with a rising cesarean delivery rate. *Am J Obstet Gynecol.* 2005; 192(1): 102-8.

– Giacalone P, Daures J, Vignal J, et al. Pfannenstiel versus Maylard incision for cesarean delivery. *Obstet Gynecol.* 2002; 99(5 Pt 1): 745-50.

– Glezerman M. Five years to the term breech trial: the rise and fall of a randomized controlled trial. *Am J Obstet Gynecol.* 2006; 194(1): 20-5.

– Gottlieb A, Galan H. Shoulder dystocia: an update. *Obstet Gynecol Clin North Am.* 2007; 34(3): 501-31.

– Grobman W, Gersnoviez R, Landon M, et al. Pregnancy outcomes for women with placenta previa in relation to the number of prior cesarean deliveries. *Obstet Gynecol.* 2007; 110(6): 1249-55.

– Grootscholten K, Kok M, Oei S, et al. External cephalic version-related risks: a meta-analysis. *Obstet Gynecol.* 2008; 112(5): 1143-51.

– Gyamfi C, Juhasz G, Gyamfi P, et al. Single- versus double-layer uterine incision closure and uterine rupture. *J Matern Fetal Neonatal Med.* 2006; 19(10): 639-43.

– Hamilton B, Martin J, Sutton P. Births: preliminary data for 2003. *Natl Vital Stat Rep.* 2004; 53(9): 1-17.

– Hankins G, Clark S, Munn M. Cesarean section on request at 39 weeks: impact on shoulder dystocia, fetal trauma, neonatal encephalopathy, and intrauterine fetal demise. *Semin Perinatol.* 2006; 30(5): 276-87.

– Hannah M, Hannah W, Hewson S, et al. Planned caesarean section versus planned vaginal birth for breech presentation at term: a randomised multicentre trial. Term Breech Trial Collaborative Group. *Lancet.* 2000; 356(9239): 1375-83.

– Harper M, Byington R, Espeland M, et al. Pregnancy-related death and health care services. *Obstet Gynecol.* 2003; 102(2): 273-8.

– Harrigill K, Miller H, Haynes D. The effect of intraabdominal irrigation at cesarean delivery on maternal morbidity. *Obstet Gynecol.* 2003; 101(1): 80-5.

– Heit J, Kobbervig C, James A, et al. Trends in the incidence of venous thromboembolism during pregnancy or postpartum: a 30-year population-based study. *Ann Intern Med.* 2005; 143(10): 697-706.

– Hellums E, Lin M, Ramsey P. Prophylactic subcutaneous drainage for prevention of wound complications after cesarean delivery--a metaanalysis. *Am J Obstet Gynecol.* 2007; 197(3): 229-35.

– Hofmeyr G, Mathai M, Shah A, et al. Techniques for caesarean section. *Cochrane Database Syst Rev.* 2008; CD004662.

– Hohlagschwandtner M, Ruecklinger E, Husslein P, et al. Is the formation of a bladder flap at cesarean necessary? A randomized trial. *Obstet Gynecol.* 2001; 98(6): 1089-92.

– Homer C, Kurinczuk J, Spark P, et al. Planned vaginal delivery or planned caesarean delivery in women with extreme obesity. *BJOG.* 2011; 118(4): 480-7.

– How H, Harris B, Pietrantoni M, et al. Is vaginal delivery preferable to elective cesarean delivery in fetuses with a known ventral wall defect? *Am J Obstet Gynecol.* 2000; 182(6): 1527-34.

– Landon M. Cesarean section. Gabbe S, Niebyl J, Simpson J, eds. *Obstetrics.* 5th ed. New York, NY: Churchill Livingston; 2007.

– Landon M. Vaginal birth after cesarean delivery. *Clin Perinatol.* 2008; 35(3): 491-504.

– Lee Y, D'Alton M. Cesarean delivery on maternal request: maternal and neonatal complications. *Curr Opin Obstet Gynecol.* 2008; 20(6): 597-601.

– Levy R, Chernomoretz T, Appelman Z, et al. Head pushing versus reverse breech extraction in cases of impacted fetal head during Cesarean section. *Eur J Obstet Gynecol Reprod Biol.* 2005; 121(1): 24-6.

– Li L, Wen J, Wang L, et al. Is routine indwelling catheterisation of the bladder for caesarean section necessary? A systematic review. *BJOG*. 2011; 118(4): 400-9.

– MacDorman M, Menacker F, Declercq E. Cesarean birth in the United States: epidemiology, trends, and outcomes. *Clin Perinatol*. 2008; 35(2): 293-307.

– Mackeen A, Packard R, Ota E, et al. Timing of intravenous prophylactic antibiotics for preventing postpartum infectious morbidity in women undergoing cesarean delivery. *Cochrane Database Syst Rev*. 2014; CD009516.

– MacKenzie I, Cooke I. What is a reasonable time from decision-to-delivery by caesarean section? Evidence from 415 deliveries. *BJOG*. 2002; 109(5): 498-504.

– Martin J, Hamilton B, Sutton P, et al. Births: final data for 2002. *Natl Vital Stat Rep*. 2003; 52(10): 1-113.

– Mehta S, Bujold E, Blackwell S, et al. Is abnormal labor associated with shoulder dystocia in nulliparous women? *Am J Obstet Gynecol*. 2004. 190(6): 1604-7.

– Menacker F. Trends in cesarean rates for first births and repeat cesarean rates for low-risk women: United States, 1990-2003. *Natl Vital Stat Rep*. 2005; 54(4): 1-8.

– Moertl M, Friedrich S, Kraschl J, et al. Haemodynamic effects of carbetocin and oxytocin given as intravenous bolus on women undergoing caesarean delivery: a randomised trial. *BJOG*. 2011; 118(11): 1349-56.

– Morales M, Ceysens G, Jastrow N, et al. Spontaneous delivery or manual removal of the placenta during caesarean section: a randomised controlled trial. *BJOG*. 2004; 111(9): 908-12.

– Nelson R, Furner S, Westercamp M, et al. Cesarean delivery for the prevention of anal incontinence. *Cochrane Database Syst Rev*. 2010; CD006756.

– NIH State-of-the-Science Conference: Cesarean Delivery on Maternal Request; Bethesda, Md. NIH Consens Sci Statements. 2006; 23(1): 1-29.

– Orji E, Olabode T, Kuti O, et al. A randomised controlled trial of early initiation of oral feeding after CS. *J Matern Fetal Neonatal Med.* 2009; 22(1): 65-71.

– Patolia D, Hilliard R, Toy E, et al. Early feeding after cesarean: randomized trial. *Obstet Gynecol.* 2001; 98(1): 113-6.

– Preis K, Swiatkowska-Freund M, Janczewska I. Spina bifida--a follow-up study of neonates born from 1991 to 2001. *J Perinat Med.* 2005; 33(4): 353-6.

– Ramsey P, White A, Guinn D, et al. Subcutaneous tissue reapproximation, alone or in combination with drain, in obese women undergoing cesarean delivery. *Obstet Gynecol.* 2005; 105(5 Pt 1): 967-73.

– Rouse D, Hirtz D, Thom E, et al. A randomized, controlled trial of magnesium sulfate for the prevention of cerebral palsy. *N Engl J Med.* 2008; 359(9): 895-905.

– Rousseau J, Girard K, Turcot-Lemay L, et al. A randomized study comparing skin closure in cesarean sections: staples vs subcuticular sutures. *Am J Obstet Gynecol.* 2009; 200(3): 265.e1-4.

– Ruys T, Cornette J, Roos-Hesselink J. Pregnancy and delivery in cardiac disease. *J Cardiol.* 2013; 61(2): 107-12.

– Salihu H, Emusu D, Aliyu Z, et al. Mode of delivery and neonatal survival of infants with isolated gastroschisis. *Obstet Gynecol.* 2004; 104(4): 678-83.

– Smaill F, Gyte G. Antibiotic prophylaxis versus no prophylaxis for preventing infection after cesarean section. *Cochrane Database Syst Rev.* 2010; CD007482.

– Sung J, Daniels K, Brodzinsky L, et al. Cesarean delivery outcomes after a prolonged second stage of labor. *Am J Obstet Gynecol.* 2007; 197(3): 306.e1-5.

– Tan P, Norazilah M, Omar S. Hospital discharge on the first compared with the second day after a planned cesarean delivery: a randomized controlled trial. *Obstet Gynecol.* 2012; 120 (6): 1273-82.

– Tipton A, Cohen S, Chelmow D. Wound infection in the obese pregnant woman. *Semin Perinatol*. 2011; 35(6): 345-9.

– Tita A, Hauth J, Grimes A, et al. Decreasing incidence of postcesarean endometritis with extended-spectrum antibiotic prophylaxis. *Obstet Gynecol*. 2008; 111(1): 51-6.

– Tita A, Landon M, Spong C, et al. Timing of elective repeat cesarean delivery at term and neonatal outcomes. *N Engl J Med*. 2009; 360(2): 111-20.

– Todman D. A history of caesarean section: from ancient world to the modern era. *Aust N Z J Obstet Gynaecol*. 2007; 47(5): 357-61.

– Tuuli M, Rampersad R, Carbone J, et al. Staples compared with subcuticular suture for skin closure after cesarean delivery: a systematic review and meta-analysis. *Obstet Gynecol*. 2011; 117(3): 682-90.

– Villar J, Valladares E, Wojdyla D, et al. Caesarean delivery rates and pregnancy outcomes: the 2005 WHO global survey on maternal and perinatal health in Latin America. *Lancet*. 2006; 367(9525): 1819-29.

– Weiner Z, Ben-Shlomo I, Beck-Fruchter R, et al. Clinical and ultrasonographic weight estimation in large for gestational age fetus. *Eur J Obstet Gynecol Reprod Biol*. 2002; 105(1): 20-4.

– Yuan C, Gaskins A, Blaine A, et al. Association between Cesarean Birth and Risk of Obesity in Offspring in Childhood, Adolescence, and Early Adulthood. *JAMA Pediatr*. 2016; e162385.

www.ingramcontent.com/pod-product-compliance
Lightning Source LLC
Chambersburg PA
CBHW071254170526
45165CB00003B/1346